Living a Long and Healthy Life

The Journey of Longevity

By Clay Sherman

Kimball & Bradley Publishing

TABLE OF CONTENTS

CHAPTER 1: THE QUEST FOR LONGEVITY

Since time immemorial, the pursuit of longevity has captivated human imagination. From mythical elixirs of immortality to modern scientific breakthroughs, the quest for a longer life has been a driving force behind human endeavors, shaping cultures, philosophies, and scientific advancements. This journey through time will explore the multifaceted history of humanity's pursuit of longevity, delving into the ancient wisdom, folklore, and scientific discoveries that have shaped our understanding of aging and life extension.

ANCIENT ROOTS AND MYTHICAL ELIXIRS

The yearning for a longer life can be traced back to the earliest records of human civilization. Ancient cultures across the globe harbored beliefs in mythical elixirs, rituals, and practices that promised immortality or extended life spans. In Chinese mythology, the search for the elixir of life led to the concept of the "Peaches of Immortality," symbolic of eternal youth. Similarly, in Indian folklore, the concept of "Amrita," the nectar of immortality, emerged as a central theme.

Ancient Egyptians revered their pharaohs as god-kings, and the quest for life after death was closely linked to their search for longevity. Intricate burial practices, mummification, and the construction of elaborate tombs were all attempts to ensure an everlasting existence beyond the earthly realm.

Alchemy, often dismissed as pseudoscience today, played a significant role in the historical pursuit of longevity. Alchemists of the Middle Ages sought the philosopher's stone, believed to hold the secret to transmuting base metals into gold and achieving eternal life. These pursuits, while rooted in mysticism, laid the groundwork for the scientific exploration of life extension.

Religious Traditions and Ethical Considerations

Religious and philosophical traditions have also contributed to the discourse on longevity. Concepts of an afterlife, reincarnation, and the preservation of the soul have driven humanity's search for meaning and purpose beyond mere mortal existence. Christianity, Islam, Buddhism, and other major religions have addressed questions of mortality and offered varying perspectives on the significance of life extension.

Yet, these religious beliefs have also raised ethical dilemmas. The tension between desiring a longer life and adhering to spiritual teachings that emphasize the transient nature of life has sparked debates about the morality of pursuing immortality. The intricate interplay between faith, science, and the human condition continues to influence our perceptions of longevity.

Scientific Endeavors and Breakthroughs

The transition from mythical and mystical pursuits to a more scientific understanding of longevity began during the Enlightenment. Pioneers like Paracelsus and Robert Boyle laid the foundation for experimental methodologies, sparking a shift from alchemy to the early days of chemistry. This shift marked the dawn of a new era in which human longevity could be explored through rational inquiry.

In the 18th and 19th centuries, advances in medicine and public health started to extend average life spans. Innovations such as the smallpox vaccine, sanitation reforms, and improved hygiene led to significant reductions in mortality rates. The burgeoning field of gerontology emerged, focusing on the study of aging and its impact on health.

The 20th century witnessed a surge in scientific breakthroughs that furthered our understanding of aging and longevity. The discovery of DNA's structure by Watson and Crick in 1953 paved the way for the unraveling of genetic codes related to aging and disease. Theories like the Hayflick limit, which suggests that human cells have a finite capacity to divide, deepened our comprehension of cellular aging.

MODERN APPROACHES: CALORIC RESTRICTION, TELOMERES, AND BEYOND

In recent decades, researchers have explored a multitude of avenues to extend human life spans. Caloric restriction, a practice rooted in ancient wisdom, has been extensively studied in animal models, showing promising effects on increasing lifespan. Similarly, the study of telomeres, the protective caps on the ends of chromosomes, has uncovered their role in cellular aging and potential implications for life extension.

Advancements in biotechnology have ushered in an era of unprecedented possibilities. Gene editing technologies like CRISPR-Cas9 hold promise for eliminating disease-causing mutations and delaying the aging process. Senescence, the process of biological aging, is being targeted at the cellular level, with researchers working to develop interventions that could mitigate its effects.

ETHICAL CONSIDERATIONS AND SOCIETAL IMPLICATIONS

As the scientific community inches closer to potential breakthroughs in life extension, ethical questions loom large. The prospect of significantly prolonging life raises complex issues related to population growth, resource allocation, and quality of life. The disparity between those who could afford life-extending treatments and those who cannot creates ethical dilemmas that demand careful consideration.

Additionally, the philosophical and psychological implications of living longer warrant examination. How might extended lifespans impact our sense of purpose, relationships, and personal growth? Could the fear of death be replaced by a new set of existential concerns?

The quest for longevity has been a constant thread throughout human history, weaving its way through ancient myths, religious doctrines, and scientific exploration. From alchemical pursuits to cutting-edge biotechnology, the human drive to understand and extend life has shaped our cultures, philosophies, and collective aspirations.

As we stand at the crossroads of unprecedented scientific possibilities, the quest for longevity remains deeply intertwined with questions of ethics, identity, and purpose. The history of this endeavor underscores the complexity of human nature, our yearning for meaning, and our relentless pursuit of a future where the boundaries of age may be pushed further than ever before. In our ongoing exploration of life and its extension, may we find a harmonious balance between the wisdom of our past and the potential of our future.

In the tapestry of human desires, the longing for extended and healthier lives stands as one of the most profound threads. The quest to transcend the boundaries of mortality and bask in the glory of longevity has been an enduring pursuit throughout history. Delving into the intricate motivations that propel humanity's yearning for increased lifespan and well-being unveils a complex interplay of cultural, psychological, and personal factors that shape our aspirations. From the preservation of cherished moments to the pursuit of scientific advancements, let us embark on a journey to understand why people wish to live longer, healthier lives.

PRESERVING PRECIOUS MOMENTS

One of the most poignant reasons people seek longevity is rooted in the desire to cherish life's most precious moments. The tapestry of human existence is woven with connections and experiences that accumulate over time. The prospect of living longer provides an opportunity to witness the unfolding chapters of one's life, from the birth of children to the celebration of milestones and the deepening of relationships. The sentiment of not wanting to miss out on the joys and sorrows that life brings, of witnessing the growth and evolution of oneself and loved ones, is a profound motivation.

Cultural and Societal Influences

Cultural norms and societal expectations exert a significant influence on the desire for extended life spans. In many societies, elders are revered for their wisdom and experience, and their stories carry the legacy of generations. The cultural value placed on longevity often translates into a personal aspiration to contribute to one's family, community, or culture over an extended period. The idea of leaving a lasting impact, passing down traditions, and being a guiding presence for future generations serves as a driving force for the pursuit of a longer life.

The Fear of Regret and Unfulfilled Dreams

Regret, like a shadow cast upon the twilight of life, is a potent motivator for seeking a longer and healthier existence. The fear of reaching the end of one's journey with unfulfilled dreams and unexplored possibilities can be a powerful catalyst for action. This fear encourages individuals to seek out new experiences, take risks, and make choices that align with their passions and aspirations. The quest for longevity becomes a means to ensure that life is lived to the fullest, without the haunting specter of missed opportunities.

Scientific Advancements and Curiosity

The human spirit is intrinsically curious, and this curiosity fuels the quest for scientific advancements that can extend life and well-being. The pursuit of breakthroughs in medicine, genetics, and biotechnology reflects a deep-seated yearning to conquer the mysteries of aging and enhance the quality of life. As scientific knowledge expands, individuals are drawn to the possibility of reaping the benefits of cutting-edge innovations that promise not only a longer life but also a healthier and more vibrant one.

Human Resilience and the Drive for Survival

Embedded within the fabric of human nature is an innate drive for survival and resilience. Throughout history, humans have demonstrated remarkable adaptability in the face of challenges, be they natural disasters, plagues, or adversities. This innate resilience often translates into a profound desire to overcome the limitations of mortality. The aspiration to prolong life can be seen as an extension of humanity's intrinsic will to survive, thrive, and triumph over adversity.

SENSE OF ACCOMPLISHMENT AND LEGACY

The desire to leave a lasting legacy is a recurrent theme in the pursuit of longevity. Individuals strive to create a meaningful impact on the world, whether through their work, art, philanthropy, or other endeavors. Living longer allows for the accumulation of achievements and contributions, shaping a narrative of significance that extends beyond one's own lifetime. This sense of accomplishment and the yearning to make a mark on history often drive people to embrace the possibility of a prolonged existence.

EMBRACING EVOLVING RELATIONSHIPS

The relationships we forge throughout our lives hold a special place in our hearts. The prospect of an extended life allows for the nurturing and deepening of these relationships, fostering connections with new generations and maintaining bonds with cherished companions. The desire to witness the unfolding narratives of loved ones and to be present for the milestones and challenges they encounter plays a pivotal role in the aspiration for a longer, shared journey.

The yearning for extended and healthier lives is a fundamental human aspiration that transcends time, culture, and circumstance. From the preservation of cherished moments to the pursuit of scientific advancements, the motivations behind this quest are as diverse and intricate as the fabric of human existence itself. As we navigate the intricate interplay of cultural influences, personal aspirations, and scientific possibilities, we come to understand that the desire for longevity is a reflection of our multifaceted nature—a tapestry woven with threads of love, curiosity, resilience, and the insatiable thirst for life's myriad experiences.

In the grand tapestry of human existence, the pursuit of longevity stands as a noble aspiration. Yet, the mere passage of time is insufficient to define a life well-lived. It is in the deliberate acts of planning and goal setting that the true essence of a prolonged and meaningful existence unfolds. The art of envisioning a future, setting objectives, and working towards them holds the key to not just a longer life, but a life rich with purpose, fulfillment, and vibrancy. As we explore the intersection of planning, goal setting, and longevity, we unearth a profound connection between intentionality and the realization of a truly fulfilling journey.

Defining Longevity Beyond Time

Before delving into the reasons why planning and goal setting are crucial for longevity, it's imperative to redefine longevity itself. Longevity is not solely a measure of chronological age; rather, it's a reflection of the depth and quality of experiences one accumulates over time. Planning and goal setting align with this broader definition, as they provide the framework for carving out a life marked by intentionality, growth, and a sense of purpose. In essence, true longevity emerges not merely from a prolonged existence, but from the cultivation of a life that is actively shaped and guided.

The Role of Purpose in Prolonged Existence

One of the pivotal elements that planning and goal setting contribute to longevity is the cultivation of purpose. Studies consistently demonstrate that individuals who live with a sense of purpose tend to lead longer, healthier lives. Planning and goal setting serve as the conduits through which purpose is channeled. When individuals set meaningful objectives and outline strategies to achieve them, they infuse their lives with a profound sense of direction and meaning. This purpose-driven approach fosters a motivation to engage with life fully, thereby contributing to a longer and more fulfilling journey.

ENHANCING PSYCHOLOGICAL WELL-BEING

The mental and emotional dimensions of life play a critical role in influencing overall well-being and longevity. Planning and goal setting have been linked to enhanced psychological well-being, offering individuals a sense of control, optimism, and empowerment. The act of envisioning a future and breaking it down into actionable goals cultivates a positive mindset that transcends age. This mental resilience and adaptability become crucial in navigating the challenges and transitions that come with the passage of time.

MITIGATING THE RISK OF INACTIVITY AND STAGNATION

A life devoid of purposeful direction often leads to a state of inactivity and stagnation. As individuals age, this lack of engagement can have detrimental effects on both physical and cognitive health. Planning and goal setting counteract this by instilling a dynamic approach to life. By continuously striving towards objectives, individuals remain engaged, curious, and open to growth. The pursuit of goals keeps the mind sharp, the body active, and the spirit invigorated—attributes that are closely associated with longevity and vitality.

FOSTERING SOCIAL CONNECTIONS AND NETWORKS

Human beings are inherently social creatures, and meaningful connections with others contribute significantly to a longer and more fulfilling life. Planning and goal setting provide opportunities to forge and nurture these connections. Shared goals can become collaborative endeavors that bring individuals together, fostering a sense of community and camaraderie. This social engagement not only enhances emotional well-being but also serves as a buffer against the isolation that can sometimes accompany aging.

Adapting to Changing Circumstances

The journey of life is marked by a series of transitions and transformations. From career shifts to family dynamics, individuals constantly navigate changing circumstances. Planning and goal setting equip individuals with the tools to adapt and thrive amidst these changes. By setting flexible yet purposeful objectives, individuals can navigate transitions with resilience and a positive outlook. This adaptability becomes instrumental in maintaining a sense of agency and vitality even as circumstances evolve.

Cultivating a Legacy of Impact

The desire to leave a lasting impact on the world is a universal human aspiration. Planning and goal setting enable individuals to create a legacy that extends beyond their own lives. By setting goals aligned with their values and aspirations, individuals can contribute to their communities, families, or larger causes. This legacy of impact not only imbues life with a profound sense of purpose but also extends the ripple effects of one's existence far into the future.

Conclusion

In the grand narrative of life, the chapters are not written by chance alone. They are shaped by the intentions, aspirations, and actions of individuals who dare to envision a future and work diligently towards it. Planning and goal setting, far from being mere administrative tasks, are the architects of a life that embodies true longevity—a life marked by purpose, vibrancy, and the fulfillment of dreams. As individuals embark on this journey of intentional living, they pave the way for a prolonged existence that transcends time and resonates with the profound echoes of a life well-lived.

CHAPTER 2: EATING FOR LONGEVITY

In the pursuit of a long and vibrant life, our dietary choices play a central role. The foods we consume have the power to influence our health, well-being, and longevity. From the selection of nutrient-rich ingredients to the avoidance of harmful substances, the significance of eating for longevity cannot be overstated. This comprehensive exploration will delve into the principles of eating for longevity, encompassing what to eat, what not to eat, and the crucial distinction between adopting a lifestyle and following a diet.

The connection between what we eat and how long we live has been a subject of fascination for centuries. From ancient wisdom traditions to modern scientific research, the influence of diet on human longevity has been extensively explored. While no magical elixir of eternal life exists, the evidence consistently points to the profound impact that our dietary choices can have on our quality of life and the years we have on this planet.

In an era marked by a surplus of food options and conflicting nutritional advice, the concept of "eating for longevity" emerges as a beacon of clarity. This concept is not about deprivation or strict rules; rather, it's a philosophy that encourages us to make informed, mindful choices that nourish our bodies, fortify our health, and support the goal of living a prolonged and fulfilling life.

This chapter will take you on a journey through the essential components of eating for longevity, encompassing not only the foods that should be embraced but also those that should be limited or avoided. Furthermore, we will explore the distinction between adopting a sustainable lifestyle versus merely adhering to a temporary diet, highlighting the importance of holistic and lasting changes.

By the time you reach the conclusion of this chapter, you will have gained a thorough understanding of the principles, practices, and mindset required to make dietary choices that nurture both your present well-being and your future longevity.

The Link Between Diet and Longevity

Before delving into the specifics of what to eat and what to avoid, it's imperative to grasp the profound link between diet and longevity. Scientific research continually reinforces the notion that the foods we consume have a direct impact on our overall health and the aging process. The foods we choose can either promote inflammation, oxidative stress, and chronic diseases or act as powerful allies in the prevention of these ailments.

A balanced and nutrient-dense diet can support a range of bodily functions, including immune function, cellular repair, brain health, and cardiovascular health. Moreover, the right dietary choices can help regulate blood sugar levels, maintain a healthy weight, and optimize energy levels—factors that contribute to a vibrant and extended life.

The journey to eating for longevity is not about extreme restrictions or drastic changes overnight. Rather, it's a gradual process of adopting habits that align with the values of nourishing your body and promoting vitality.

WHAT TO EAT FOR LONGEVITY

NUTRIENT-DENSE FOODS

At the heart of eating for longevity lies the principle of consuming nutrient-dense foods. Nutrient density refers to the ratio of essential nutrients to the number of calories in a given food. This means that every bite you take should offer a substantial amount of vitamins, minerals, antioxidants, and other beneficial compounds in relation to its caloric content.

Foods that are rich in nutrients include:

Leafy Greens: Spinach, kale, Swiss chard, and other leafy greens are packed with vitamins (such as A, C, K), minerals (like iron and magnesium), and fiber.

Colorful Vegetables: Vibrant vegetables like bell peppers, carrots, and tomatoes provide a range of antioxidants and phytonutrients that support health.

Fruits: Berries, citrus fruits, apples, and other fruits offer an array of vitamins, minerals, and fiber while containing natural sugars.

Whole Grains: Whole grains like quinoa, brown rice, and whole wheat provide complex carbohydrates, fiber, and essential nutrients.

Legumes: Beans, lentils, and chickpeas are excellent sources of plant-based protein, fiber, and essential minerals.

Nuts and Seeds: Almonds, walnuts, chia seeds, and flaxseeds offer healthy fats, protein, and a variety of micronutrients.

Lean Proteins: Fish, poultry, lean meats, and plant-based protein sources (such as tofu and tempeh) contribute to muscle maintenance and overall health.

PLANT-BASED EMPHASIS

A plant-based dietary approach has gained substantial attention in recent years for its potential benefits on longevity and well-being. While this doesn't necessarily mean adopting a strict vegetarian or vegan lifestyle, incorporating a substantial portion of plant-based foods into your diet can contribute to longevity.

Plants provide an abundance of fiber, antioxidants, and phytonutrients that support digestive health, reduce inflammation, and protect against chronic diseases. In particular, the Mediterranean diet—an eating pattern rich in vegetables, fruits, whole grains, olive oil, and moderate amounts of lean proteins—has been associated with improved heart health, cognitive function, and longevity.

INCORPORATING LEAN PROTEINS

Protein is a crucial component of a balanced diet, playing a vital role in muscle maintenance, immune function, and the repair of body tissues. However, not all proteins are created equal. Lean proteins, which are low in saturated fats and devoid of processed additives, are particularly beneficial for longevity.

Opt for protein sources such as:

Fish: Fatty fish like salmon, mackerel, and sardines are rich in omega-3 fatty acids, which have been linked to heart health and cognitive function.

Poultry: Skinless poultry (chicken and turkey) provides lean protein without the excess saturated fat found in some meats.

Legumes: Beans, lentils, and other legumes are excellent plant-based sources of protein that also offer fiber and essential nutrients.

Nuts and Seeds: These options not only provide healthy fats but also contribute a moderate amount of protein to your diet.

HEALTHY FATS AND OMEGA-3S

Contrary to the outdated notion that all fats are harmful, it's important to distinguish between healthy fats and those that are detrimental to health. Healthy fats, such as monounsaturated and polyunsaturated fats, play a role in maintaining cell structure, brain health, and overall well-being.

Sources of healthy fats include:

Olive Oil: A staple of the Mediterranean diet, extra virgin olive oil is rich in monounsaturated fats and antioxidants.

Avocado: Avocados offer a creamy texture along with monounsaturated fats, vitamins, and minerals.

Nuts and Seeds: Almonds, walnuts, chia seeds, and flaxseeds provide a mix of healthy fats, protein, and essential nutrients.

Fatty Fish: As mentioned earlier, fatty fish like salmon, mackerel, and sardines are excellent sources of omega-3 fatty acids.

Omega-3 fatty acids, a type of polyunsaturated fat, are particularly noteworthy for their potential to support heart health, cognitive function, and inflammation reduction. Including fatty fish, flaxseeds, chia seeds, and walnuts in your diet can contribute to your omega-3 intake.

ANTIOXIDANT-RICH CHOICES
Antioxidants are compounds that help protect our cells from damage caused by harmful molecules called free radicals. Free radicals can contribute to oxidative stress, inflammation, and

chronic diseases. Including antioxidant-rich foods in your diet can help combat this damage and promote longevity.

Foods high in antioxidants include:

Berries: Blueberries, strawberries, raspberries, and other berries are packed with vitamins, minerals, and phytonutrients.

Dark Chocolate: Dark chocolate with a high cocoa content contains flavonoids, which have antioxidant properties.

Colorful Vegetables and Fruits: A diverse range of colorful produce provides an array of antioxidants.

Green Tea: Green tea is rich in catechins, powerful antioxidants that have been associated with various health benefits.

Spices: Turmeric, ginger, cinnamon, and other spices contain compounds with antioxidant and anti-inflammatory properties.

HYDRATION AND HERBAL TEAS
Staying well-hydrated is essential for maintaining bodily functions, supporting digestion, and promoting overall health. While water should be your primary source of hydration, herbal teas can also offer additional benefits.

Certain herbal teas, such as green tea, chamomile tea, and hibiscus tea, are known for their potential health-promoting properties. Green tea, for instance, contains catechins that have antioxidant effects. Chamomile tea may have calming and anti-inflammatory effects, while hibiscus tea has been associated with improved heart health.

What to Avoid for Longevity

Processed and Ultra-Processed Foods

In contrast to nutrient-dense whole foods, processed and ultra-processed foods are often stripped of essential nutrients and loaded with added sugars, unhealthy fats, and artificial additives. These foods include sugary snacks, sweetened beverages, fast food, and pre-packaged meals.

The consumption of processed foods has been linked to obesity, diabetes, heart disease, and other chronic health conditions. Moreover, these foods tend to be calorie-dense and lacking in the essential nutrients that support longevity.

Excessive Sugar and Sweeteners

The excessive consumption of added sugars has been identified as a major contributor to various health issues, including obesity, type 2 diabetes, and heart disease. Foods and beverages that are high in added sugars can lead to blood sugar spikes, insulin resistance, and inflammation—factors that can compromise longevity.

To reduce your sugar intake, consider:

- Limiting Sugary Drinks: Soda, fruit juices, energy drinks, and sweetened teas are often laden with added sugars.
- Reading Labels: Check nutrition labels for hidden sources of added sugars in processed foods.
- Choosing Natural Sweeteners: When needed, opt for natural sweeteners like honey, maple syrup, or stevia in moderation.

Trans Fats and Artificial Additives

Trans fats are artificial fats created through the hydrogenation process, which transforms liquid oils into solid fats. These fats are commonly found in fried foods, baked goods, and certain margarines. Trans fats are known to increase the risk of heart disease and have no place in a longevity-promoting diet.

Additionally, artificial additives such as artificial sweeteners, colors, and flavors have been associated with potential health risks. Minimizing the consumption of foods that contain these additives can contribute to a more healthful and longevity-focused diet.

RED AND PROCESSED MEATS

The consumption of red and processed meats has been a topic of debate in the context of longevity and health. The World Health Organization (WHO) has classified processed meats, such as bacon, sausages, and deli meats, as carcinogens. Red meats, particularly when prepared through high-temperature cooking methods, have also been linked to an increased risk of certain cancers.

While you don't need to eliminate these meats entirely, moderation is key. Consider leaner protein sources, such as poultry, fish, legumes, and plant-based alternatives.

HIGH SODIUM INTAKE

Excess sodium intake, often derived from salt, is associated with high blood pressure, which is a major risk factor for heart disease and stroke. Foods high in sodium include processed snacks, canned soups, fast food, and salty condiments.

To reduce sodium intake:

- Cook at Home: Preparing meals at home allows you to control the amount of salt used in your dishes.
- Choose Fresh Ingredients: Opt for fresh vegetables, fruits, and whole foods that naturally contain lower levels of sodium.
- Read Labels: Be mindful of sodium content in packaged foods and choose lower-sodium options whenever possible.

OVERCONSUMPTION OF ALCOHOL

While moderate alcohol consumption has been associated with certain health benefits, excessive drinking can lead to a range of health issues, including liver disease, cardiovascular problems, and an increased risk of accidents. To promote longevity, it's important to consume alcohol in moderation, if at all.

Moderate alcohol consumption is generally defined as up to one drink per day for women and up to two drinks per day for men. However, it's important to note that not everyone should consume alcohol, especially if there are underlying health conditions or contraindications.

THE DIFFERENCE BETWEEN A LIFESTYLE AND A DIET

A pivotal aspect of eating for longevity is recognizing and embracing the distinction between adopting a lifestyle and following a diet. While these terms are often used interchangeably, they encompass fundamentally different approaches to food and well-being.

DIET: A TEMPORARY APPROACH

Diets are typically characterized by a set of rules, restrictions, or guidelines that dictate what and how much you should eat. They often focus on short-term goals such as weight loss, and they may require significant changes in eating habits for a limited period.

Diets can provide rapid results in the short term, but they often lack sustainability. They can be challenging to maintain over time, leading to cycles of restriction, indulgence, and frustration. Many diets are also centered around deprivation and may not provide the necessary balance of nutrients to support long-term health.

LIFESTYLE: SUSTAINABLE HABITS

On the other hand, a lifestyle approach to eating is rooted in cultivating sustainable habits that promote overall well-being. Rather than focusing solely on short-term goals, a lifestyle approach considers the broader context of health, happiness, and longevity.

A lifestyle approach encompasses:

- Mindful Eating: Paying attention to hunger and fullness cues, savoring flavors, and being present during meals.
- Balanced Choices: Striving for a balanced and varied diet that includes a range of nutrients from whole foods.
- Enjoyment: Embracing foods you enjoy in moderation, without guilt or restrictions.
- Long-Term Goals: Prioritizing habits that support health and well-being over the course of your life.

MINDFUL EATING AND INTUITIVE CHOICES

Mindful eating is a cornerstone of the lifestyle approach. It involves being fully present during meals, savoring each bite, and paying attention to the body's signals of hunger and fullness. By practicing mindful eating, you can cultivate a deeper connection with your body's needs, making it easier to make choices that support your well-being.

Intuitive eating is closely aligned with mindful eating. It encourages you to trust your body's cues, honor your cravings, and make food choices based on your internal signals rather than external rules. This approach promotes a healthy relationship with food and helps prevent the cycle of restrictive dieting.

Cultural and Regional Influences

As you navigate the path of eating for longevity, it's important to recognize the cultural and regional influences that shape dietary habits and traditions. Different societies have cultivated unique approaches to eating that reflect their values, resources, and historical practices. Learning from these cultural paradigms can offer valuable insights into longevity-promoting dietary patterns.

Blue Zones: Learning from Long-Lived Communities

Blue Zones are regions around the world where a higher-than-average number of people live remarkably long and healthy lives. These regions include areas in Okinawa (Japan), Sardinia (Italy), Nicoya (Costa Rica), Ikaria (Greece), and Loma Linda (California, USA).

The dietary patterns of Blue Zone communities share several characteristics:

- Plant-Based Emphasis: Blue Zone diets are primarily plant-based, with a strong emphasis on vegetables, legumes, and whole grains.
- Moderate Meat Consumption: While meat is not entirely excluded, it's consumed in smaller quantities and often serves as a flavoring rather than a main course.
- Social Eating: Meals are often shared with family and friends, promoting social connections and a sense of community.
- Natural Foods: Processed foods are limited, and traditional cooking methods are favored over industrial food production.
- Moderation and Mindfulness: Blue Zone inhabitants tend to eat until they're 80% full, practicing mindful eating and avoiding overconsumption.
- Studying the dietary habits of Blue Zone communities can provide valuable insights into the practices that contribute to their exceptional longevity.

MEDITERRANEAN DIET: A MODEL FOR LONGEVITY

The Mediterranean diet is a well-studied and celebrated dietary pattern that has been associated with a range of health benefits and longevity. This diet is inspired by the eating habits of countries bordering the Mediterranean Sea, such as Greece, Italy, and Spain.

Key features of the Mediterranean diet include:

- Abundance of Plant-Based Foods: The diet is rich in fruits, vegetables, legumes, nuts, and whole grains.
- Olive Oil: Olive oil is a primary source of fat, providing monounsaturated fats and antioxidants.
- Moderate Fish and Poultry: Fish and poultry are consumed in moderation, while red meat is limited.
- Herbs and Spices: Herbs and spices are used for flavoring instead of excessive salt.
- Red Wine (in moderation): Some Mediterranean cultures enjoy red wine in moderation, often during meals.
- Social and Active Lifestyle: Regular physical activity and social connections are integral to the Mediterranean way of life.

The Mediterranean diet is not just about what you eat; it's a holistic lifestyle that encompasses social interactions, physical activity, and a strong connection to nature.

ASIAN TRADITIONS: BALANCE AND DIVERSITY

Asian dietary traditions vary widely across the continent, but certain principles are common to many Asian cultures. These traditions often emphasize balance, moderation, and the inclusion of a variety of foods.

Key aspects of Asian dietary traditions include:

- Plant-Based Staples: Many Asian diets center around rice, noodles, and other grains, often accompanied by vegetables and legumes.
- Lean Protein Sources: Fish, tofu, tempeh, and legumes are frequently included as sources of protein.
- Herbs and Spices: A wide range of herbs and spices are used to enhance flavor and provide potential health benefits.
- Fermented Foods: Fermented foods like kimchi, miso, and yogurt can contribute to gut health.
- Tea Consumption: Traditional teas like green tea and herbal infusions are often consumed for their potential health benefits.

THE ROLE OF MODERATION AND BALANCE

In the pursuit of longevity, the concepts of moderation and balance are essential guides. A balanced approach to eating involves making mindful choices that prioritize a wide range of nutrients while allowing for occasional treats.

ENJOYING TREATS MINDFULLY

Eating for longevity does not mean completely depriving yourself of indulgent treats. In fact, allowing yourself to enjoy foods you love in moderation can contribute to a sustainable and enjoyable eating pattern. The key is to savor these treats mindfully, paying attention to taste, texture, and satisfaction.

By incorporating treats into your diet without guilt or restriction, you can prevent the all-or-nothing mentality often associated with diets. This, in turn, promotes a healthier relationship with food and supports your overall well-being.

BALANCING NUTRITIONAL NEEDS

Balancing your nutritional needs involves ensuring that you're meeting your body's requirements for essential nutrients. Rather than focusing on strict calorie counts or specific macronutrient ratios, aim to incorporate a variety of nutrient-dense foods into your meals.

Strive for a balance of:

- Carbohydrates: Focus on whole grains, vegetables, and fruits as your primary sources of carbohydrates.
- Proteins: Include lean protein sources such as fish, poultry, legumes, and plant-based alternatives.
- Fats: Choose healthy fats from sources like avocados, nuts, seeds, and olive oil.
- Vitamins and Minerals: Prioritize a diverse range of colorful vegetables and fruits to ensure a variety of vitamins and minerals.
- Fiber: Incorporate fiber-rich foods to support digestive health and promote satiety.

EATING FOR LONGEVITY: A PERSONALIZED APPROACH

Just as each person's journey through life is unique, their approach to eating for longevity should be personalized to their individual needs, preferences, and circumstances. Factors such as genetics, age, health conditions, and activity levels all play a role in determining the optimal dietary choices for long-term well-being.

GENETIC FACTORS

Genetics can influence how your body processes and responds to different nutrients. For instance, some individuals may have a genetic predisposition to certain conditions or may metabolize nutrients differently. Genetic testing and personalized nutrition approaches can provide insights into how your unique genetic makeup can guide your dietary choices.

INDIVIDUALIZED DIETARY PREFERENCES

Eating for longevity should align with your personal tastes and preferences. If you enjoy the flavors and textures of certain foods, find ways to incorporate them into your diet in a healthful manner. This approach ensures that your eating pattern is sustainable and enjoyable over the long term.

ADAPTIVE CHANGES OVER TIME

As you journey through different stages of life, your nutritional needs and preferences may evolve. Pregnancy, aging, changes in activity levels, and shifts in health status can all impact your dietary requirements. A flexible and adaptive approach to eating ensures that you continue to prioritize your well-being as your circumstances change.

THE POWER OF MINDFUL EATING

Mindful eating is a cornerstone of the longevity-promoting lifestyle. It goes beyond the mere selection of foods and invites you to engage with eating as a sensory experience. By practicing mindful eating, you can enhance your enjoyment of meals, cultivate a positive relationship with food, and support your overall health and well-being.

SAVORING EACH BITE

Mindful eating encourages you to savor each bite, paying attention to the flavors, textures, and aromas of your food. This practice not only enhances your culinary experience but also allows you to better recognize when you're satisfied.

RECOGNIZING HUNGER AND FULLNESS

Tuning into your body's signals of hunger and fullness is a fundamental aspect of mindful eating. Rather than relying on external cues or preconceived portion sizes, trust your body to guide you in determining when to start and stop eating.

REDUCING STRESS AND EMOTIONAL EATING

Mindful eating can also help you become more attuned to emotional eating triggers. By practicing mindfulness, you can distinguish between true physical hunger and the urge to eat in response to stress, boredom, or other emotions. This awareness empowers you to address emotional eating in more healthful ways.

CONCLUSION

In the grand journey of life, the foods we choose to nourish our bodies have a profound impact on our health, well-being, and longevity. Eating for longevity is not a restrictive or temporary endeavor—it's a lifelong commitment to making informed, mindful choices that promote vitality and well-being.

The principles of eating for longevity go beyond a list of dos and don'ts. They encompass a holistic approach to nourishing your body, mind, and spirit. By embracing nutrient-dense foods, prioritizing plant-based options, and practicing mindful eating, you can create a foundation for a vibrant and prolonged life.

Remember that the journey to eating for longevity is as unique as your own fingerprint. What works best for you may differ from what works for others. It's important to cultivate a personalized approach that aligns with your preferences, needs, and circumstances.

As you embark on this path, view eating as a celebration of life—a joyful and nourishing act that supports your health and longevity. By nurturing your body and making choices that align with your values, you're investing in a future filled with vitality, purpose, and the opportunity to savor each moment to the fullest.

Chapter 3: Exercise for Longevity

The pursuit of longevity is a journey that intertwines the physical, mental, and emotional dimensions of our lives. Exercise emerges as a critical component of this journey, offering a wealth of benefits that extend far beyond the confines of a gym or a track. From reducing the risk of chronic diseases to enhancing mental well-being, exercise has the remarkable power to sculpt a life marked by vitality, strength, and resilience.

In an era where sedentary lifestyles have become the norm and modern conveniences have minimized physical exertion, the importance of exercise for longevity cannot be overstated. This comprehensive guide will serve as your compass, navigating the vast landscape of exercise options, providing guidance on how to start, what to do, and what to avoid in order to ensure a purposeful and sustainable path towards health and vitality.

The Link Between Exercise and Longevity

Before delving into the specifics of exercise for longevity, it's crucial to understand the profound link between physical activity and an extended, high-quality life. Scientific research consistently demonstrates that regular exercise is associated with a range of health benefits that contribute to longevity:

- Heart Health: Exercise strengthens the heart muscle, improves circulation, and reduces the risk of cardiovascular diseases such as heart attacks and strokes.
- Weight Management: Physical activity helps maintain a healthy weight by burning calories and promoting muscle mass, which, in turn, boosts metabolism.
- Bone Health: Weight-bearing exercises like walking, jogging, and resistance training support bone density and reduce the risk of osteoporosis.

- Mental Well-Being: Exercise releases endorphins, which are natural mood elevators that combat stress, anxiety, and depression.
- Cognitive Function: Physical activity has been linked to improved cognitive function, memory, and reduced risk of cognitive decline.
- Blood Sugar Regulation: Regular exercise improves insulin sensitivity and helps regulate blood sugar levels, reducing the risk of type 2 diabetes.
- Immune System Support: Moderate exercise enhances immune function, making the body more resilient against infections and illnesses.
- Joint Health: Engaging in appropriate exercises can help maintain joint flexibility, reduce stiffness, and alleviate discomfort.

How to Start Exercising for Longevity

Embarking on a journey of exercise for longevity requires a thoughtful and strategic approach. Starting gradually, setting realistic goals, and finding activities you enjoy are all essential elements of a successful and sustainable exercise routine.

Assessing Your Current Fitness Level

Before diving into any exercise routine, it's important to assess your current fitness level. This assessment helps you understand your strengths, limitations, and areas that may need improvement. Consider factors such as your cardiovascular endurance, muscular strength, flexibility, and balance.

Setting Realistic Goals

Setting achievable goals is key to staying motivated and on track. Goals can be both short-term and long-term, such as aiming to walk for 30 minutes a day or completing a 5K race. Realistic goals ensure that you don't overwhelm yourself and set the stage for gradual progress.

Incorporating Variety and Enjoyment

Variety is the spice of life, and it applies to exercise as well. Engaging in a variety of activities not only prevents boredom but also ensures that different muscle groups are targeted and that you're receiving a well-rounded fitness experience. Choose activities that you genuinely enjoy, whether it's dancing, hiking, swimming, or practicing yoga.

Starting Slowly and Gradually Increasing Intensity

When starting an exercise routine, the temptation to dive in with intensity can be strong. However, beginning slowly and gradually increasing the intensity is crucial for preventing injuries and overexertion. This approach allows your body to adapt and build a strong foundation before taking on more challenging workouts.

What Types of Exercise to Do for Longevity

A well-rounded exercise routine encompasses a variety of components, each offering unique benefits for longevity and overall well-being.

Cardiovascular Exercise

Cardiovascular exercise, often referred to as "cardio," involves activities that elevate your heart rate and improve cardiovascular health. These exercises increase your lung capacity, strengthen the heart, and promote efficient oxygen delivery throughout the body.

Examples of cardiovascular exercises include:

- **Walking:** A simple yet effective form of exercise that can be done almost anywhere.
- **Running:** More intense than walking, running improves cardiovascular fitness and burns calories.
- **Cycling:** Whether outdoors or on a stationary bike, cycling is great for lower body strength and endurance.

- **Swimming:** A low-impact exercise that engages multiple muscle groups and enhances cardiovascular health.
- **Dancing:** A fun and creative way to get your heart pumping while enjoying music and movement.

STRENGTH TRAINING

Strength training, also known as resistance training, focuses on building and toning muscles. It plays a critical role in maintaining lean body mass, boosting metabolism, and enhancing functional strength for daily activities.

Strength training exercises include:

- **Bodyweight Exercises:** Push-ups, squats, lunges, and planks are effective bodyweight exercises that require no equipment.
- **Weight Lifting:** Using dumbbells, barbells, or resistance bands, weight lifting targets specific muscle groups for increased strength.
- **Resistance Machines:** Available at gyms, resistance machines provide controlled movements to target various muscle groups.

FLEXIBILITY AND BALANCE EXERCISES

Flexibility and balance exercises are often overlooked but are crucial for maintaining joint health, preventing falls, and promoting overall mobility.

Examples of flexibility and balance exercises include:

- **Yoga:** Yoga combines flexibility, balance, and mindfulness, enhancing both physical and mental well-being.
- **Pilates:** Similar to yoga, Pilates focuses on core strength, flexibility, and posture.
- **Tai Chi:** An ancient practice that improves balance, coordination, and relaxation through slow, flowing movements.

MIND-BODY PRACTICES

Mind-body practices combine physical movement with mental focus and relaxation. These exercises not only promote physical health but also enhance mental clarity and emotional well-being.

Mind-body practices include:

- **Yoga:** As mentioned earlier, yoga blends physical postures with breath awareness and meditation.
- **Pilates:** Alongside its physical benefits, Pilates emphasizes mindfulness, concentration, and breath control.
- **Tai Chi:** With its emphasis on meditation in motion, Tai Chi cultivates a sense of inner calm and mindfulness.

AVOIDING COMMON EXERCISE MISTAKES

As you embark on your exercise journey, it's important to be aware of common mistakes that can hinder progress and potentially lead to injuries.

OVERTRAINING AND BURNOUT

Overenthusiasm can lead to overtraining, which can have detrimental effects on your body. Overtraining not only increases the risk of injury but can also lead to burnout, fatigue, and decreased motivation. It's important to prioritize rest and recovery, allowing your body to repair and adapt to the physical stress of exercise.

NEGLECTING PROPER FORM AND TECHNIQUE

Proper form and technique are essential to prevent injuries and optimize the benefits of exercise. Performing exercises with incorrect form can strain muscles, joints, and ligaments. If you're new to a particular exercise, consider seeking guidance from a qualified fitness professional to ensure you're using the correct form.

IGNORING REST AND RECOVERY

Rest and recovery are vital components of any exercise routine. Your body requires time to heal and rebuild after workouts. Neglecting rest can lead to overtraining, fatigue, and impaired performance. Incorporate rest days into your routine and listen to your body's signals for when to take a break.

Focusing Solely on Intensity

While high-intensity workouts can be effective, they shouldn't be the sole focus of your exercise routine. Balance your routine with a variety of intensity levels, including low- and moderate-intensity exercises. Mixing different types of exercises and intensity levels can reduce the risk of burnout and provide a more well-rounded approach to fitness.

The Role of Lifestyle Factors

Exercise is just one piece of the puzzle when it comes to longevity. Lifestyle factors, such as nutrition, sleep, stress management, and social connections, all play interconnected roles in supporting your overall well-being.

Nutrition and Hydration

Proper nutrition is essential for fueling your body and supporting your exercise efforts. A balanced diet rich in whole foods provides the nutrients your body needs to perform at its best. Hydration is equally important, as staying properly hydrated enhances your energy levels and supports various bodily functions.

Sleep and Stress Management

Quality sleep is crucial for muscle recovery, hormone regulation, and overall health. Prioritize getting enough restful sleep to support your exercise routine. Additionally, managing stress through relaxation techniques, mindfulness, and other stress-reduction strategies can improve your mental and emotional well-being.

Social Connections and Support

Engaging in physical activity with others can provide motivation, accountability, and a sense of community. Whether through group classes, sports teams, or workout buddies, social connections can make exercise more enjoyable and sustainable.

CREATING A SUSTAINABLE EXERCISE ROUTINE

Consistency is key to reaping the benefits of exercise for longevity. Creating a sustainable routine involves several important factors.

SETTING A CONSISTENT SCHEDULE

Establishing a consistent exercise schedule helps integrate physical activity into your daily routine. Consistency reduces the likelihood of skipping workouts and ensures that exercise becomes a natural part of your day.

ADAPTING TO CHANGING CIRCUMSTANCES

Life is dynamic, and circumstances change. Your exercise routine may need to adapt to factors such as changes in work schedule, family commitments, or health conditions. Instead of viewing these changes as obstacles, find creative ways to modify your routine while staying committed to your goals.

LISTENING TO YOUR BODY

Your body provides valuable feedback during exercise. Pay attention to how you feel before, during, and after workouts. If you experience pain, discomfort, or extreme fatigue, it's essential to listen to your body and make adjustments as needed.

MINDSET AND MOTIVATION

A positive mindset and intrinsic motivation are vital for maintaining a lifelong exercise routine.

CULTIVATING A POSITIVE ATTITUDE

Approach exercise with a positive attitude and a focus on the benefits it brings to your health and well-being. Cultivate a mindset that views physical activity as a gift to your body rather than a chore.

CELEBRATING PROGRESS AND SMALL WINS

Celebrate your progress, no matter how small. Each step forward is a testament to your dedication and hard work. Recognizing your achievements can boost your motivation and reinforce the positive impact of exercise.

FINDING INTRINSIC MOTIVATION

Intrinsic motivation—motivation that comes from within—is a powerful driving force. Instead of solely focusing on external factors like appearance, tap into your inner motivations, such as improved energy levels, enhanced mood, or the joy of movement.

A LIFELONG APPROACH TO EXERCISE

Exercise for longevity is not a short-term endeavor; it's a commitment to a lifelong journey of health and vitality.

EMBRACING AGING AND ADAPTATION

As you age, your exercise routine may evolve. Embrace the natural changes that come with aging and adjust your workouts to accommodate your body's changing needs. Activities like gentle yoga, water aerobics, and walking can provide lifelong benefits.

SETTING NEW GOALS AND CHALLENGES

Continually setting new goals and challenges keeps your exercise routine fresh and exciting. Whether it's aiming to run a longer distance, lift heavier weights, or try a new fitness class, setting goals encourages growth and progress.

CONCLUSION

Exercise for longevity is a profound journey that goes beyond physical appearance—it's about nurturing your body, mind, and spirit. Regular physical activity has the potential to enhance your well-being, prevent chronic diseases, and cultivate a sense of vitality that enriches every aspect of life.

As you embark on this journey, remember that exercise is not a burden; it's a gift you give to yourself. Approach it with curiosity, positivity, and a commitment to long-term well-being. By incorporating a variety of exercises, practicing self-care, and adopting a mindset of growth, you're investing in a future marked by health, strength, and an enduring zest for life. So lace up those sneakers, find activities you enjoy, and embark on a journey of exercise for longevity—one step at a time.

Chapter 4: The Longevity Mindset

The quest for longevity is a journey that extends beyond the physical realm. While exercise, nutrition, and healthy habits are pivotal, they are deeply intertwined with the power of mindset. The longevity mindset transcends the boundaries of positive thinking and encompasses a way of life that nurtures mental resilience, emotional well-being, and spiritual fulfillment. It's about embracing the present moment, cultivating gratitude, and fostering a sense of purpose that propels us toward a long and thriving existence.

The concept of the longevity mindset acknowledges that our thoughts, emotions, and beliefs are integral components of our overall health. It recognizes that the way we navigate challenges, celebrate successes, and find meaning in our lives contributes to the tapestry of our longevity journey.

The Power of Mindset

Mindset is the lens through which we perceive and interact with the world. It shapes our attitudes, influences our choices, and impacts our overall well-being. Research in the field of positive psychology has revealed that our mindset can significantly influence our physical health, mental health, and overall quality of life.

Two primary types of mindsets often come into play: a fixed mindset and a growth mindset. A fixed mindset believes that qualities and abilities are static, while a growth mindset believes that talents and skills can be developed through effort and learning. Embracing a growth mindset is closely linked to resilience, adaptability, and a willingness to face challenges as opportunities for growth.

The Longevity Mindset: A Holistic Approach

The longevity mindset is a multidimensional approach that encompasses various aspects of mental, emotional, and spiritual well-being.

MENTAL RESILIENCE

Mental resilience is the ability to navigate life's challenges with a sense of equanimity and adaptability. It involves developing coping strategies, problem-solving skills, and the capacity to bounce back from setbacks. Resilience is not about avoiding difficult situations; it's about facing them with a sense of inner strength and a belief that you have the resources to overcome them.

EMOTIONAL WELL-BEING

Emotional well-being involves recognizing and managing our emotions in a healthy way. It's about cultivating self-awareness, emotional intelligence, and the ability to regulate our feelings. Embracing the longevity mindset means acknowledging that emotions are an integral part of the human experience and that they can be harnessed to enhance our well-being.

SPIRITUAL FULFILLMENT

Spiritual fulfillment doesn't necessarily refer to religious beliefs; rather, it's about finding meaning, purpose, and connection in life. Whether through personal beliefs, values, or a sense of interconnectedness, spiritual fulfillment provides a sense of direction and purpose that adds depth and richness to our lives.

CULTIVATING THE LONGEVITY MINDSET

Cultivating the longevity mindset is an ongoing practice that involves intentional efforts to shape your thoughts, beliefs, and attitudes.

SELF-AWARENESS AND REFLECTION

Self-awareness is the foundation of personal growth. Take time to reflect on your thoughts, feelings, and reactions. This practice allows you to identify patterns, strengths, and areas that may require attention. Self-awareness also enables you to make conscious choices that align with your values and well-being.

Gratitude and Positivity

Practicing gratitude involves acknowledging and appreciating the positive aspects of life. This simple yet profound practice has been linked to improved mood, enhanced relationships, and increased overall well-being. Embracing positivity doesn't mean denying challenges; it means choosing to focus on what is going well.

Stress Management and Resilience

Stress is an inevitable part of life, but how we respond to it can significantly impact our health. Developing healthy coping mechanisms, such as mindfulness, deep breathing, and relaxation techniques, empowers you to manage stress effectively. Building resilience involves viewing challenges as opportunities for growth and developing the confidence to navigate them.

Meaning and Purpose

Finding meaning and purpose is a deeply personal journey. It involves exploring your passions, values, and the impact you want to make in the world. Having a sense of purpose can provide direction, motivation, and a profound connection to something greater than yourself.

The Impact of the Longevity Mindset on Health

The longevity mindset has a ripple effect on various dimensions of health and well-being.

Stress Reduction and Immune Health

Chronic stress can weaken the immune system and contribute to the development of various health issues. By adopting a longevity mindset that prioritizes stress management and resilience, you're enhancing your body's ability to combat stress-related negative impacts.

COGNITIVE HEALTH AND BRAIN LONGEVITY

A positive mindset has been associated with better cognitive function and a reduced risk of cognitive decline. Engaging in activities that challenge your brain, practicing mindfulness, and embracing a growth mindset can contribute to cognitive health and longevity.

PHYSICAL HEALTH AND LONGEVITY

Our beliefs and attitudes can impact physical health outcomes. A positive mindset has been linked to lower blood pressure, reduced risk of heart disease, and improved overall health. By fostering a longevity mindset, you're supporting your body's resilience and promoting optimal well-being.

SOCIAL CONNECTIONS AND EMOTIONAL HEALTH

A longevity mindset can positively influence your relationships and emotional well-being. Embracing positivity, gratitude, and empathy enhances your social interactions and contributes to a supportive network of connections—a crucial factor for mental and emotional health.

EMBRACING AGING WITH A POSITIVE PERSPECTIVE

As we age, our mindset plays a pivotal role in how we approach the changes and challenges that come with aging.

REDEFINING AGING

Embracing the longevity mindset involves redefining aging as a phase of life filled with opportunities, growth, and wisdom. It's about challenging societal stereotypes and recognizing the value that comes with accumulated life experience.

EMBRACING CHANGES AND CHALLENGES

A positive perspective on aging involves acknowledging the changes that come with the passing years and approaching them with grace and adaptability. Embracing a growth mindset allows you to view challenges as opportunities for personal evolution and resilience.

PRACTICAL STRATEGIES FOR NURTURING THE LONGEVITY MINDSET

Cultivating the longevity mindset requires deliberate and consistent practices that align with your values and well-being.

MINDFULNESS AND MEDITATION

Mindfulness and meditation are powerful tools for cultivating present-moment awareness and enhancing emotional regulation. Engaging in mindfulness practices allows you to observe your thoughts without judgment, reducing stress and promoting a sense of calm.

POSITIVE AFFIRMATIONS AND SELF-TALK

Positive affirmations and self-talk involve consciously choosing uplifting and empowering statements to counter negative thoughts. By nurturing positive self-talk, you're reinforcing a mindset of self-compassion and self-belief.

SURROUNDING YOURSELF WITH POSITIVITY

Surrounding yourself with positive influences—whether through relationships, media, or environment—creates an ecosystem that supports your longevity mindset. Choose to engage with people, activities, and content that uplift and inspire you.

ENGAGING IN LIFELONG LEARNING

A growth mindset thrives on continuous learning and personal development. Embrace opportunities to expand your knowledge, acquire new skills, and explore areas of interest. Lifelong learning not only keeps your mind sharp but also fosters a sense of curiosity and engagement with life.

TRANSCENDING OBSTACLES AND ADVERSITY

The longevity mindset equips you with tools to transcend obstacles and navigate adversity with resilience and grace.

HARNESSING RESILIENCE DURING DIFFICULT TIMES

During challenging times, resilience empowers you to cope, adapt, and eventually thrive. Drawing on your well-cultivated resilience, you're able to face adversity with a sense of determination and an unwavering belief in your ability to overcome.

TURNING SETBACKS INTO OPPORTUNITIES FOR GROWTH
A setback is not a permanent state but a momentary detour on your journey. By embracing the longevity mindset, setbacks become opportunities for growth, learning, and evolving into a stronger version of yourself.

CONCLUSION

The longevity mindset is a holistic approach to life that recognizes the intricate connection between mind, body, and spirit. It's about embracing a growth mindset, fostering mental resilience, and nurturing emotional well-being. As you cultivate this mindset, you're investing in a life marked by vitality, purpose, and an enduring zest for growth.

The journey of nurturing the longevity mindset is ongoing—an evolving dance between self-awareness, gratitude, resilience, and learning. As you navigate the complexities of life, remember that your mindset is a powerful compass that guides you toward a flourishing and purposeful existence. Embrace the challenges, celebrate the triumphs, and embark on a lifelong journey of well-being that enriches every facet of your being.

CHAPTER 5: LONGEVITY AND YOUR CAREER

Our career choices are not only instrumental in shaping our professional lives but also exert a profound influence on our overall well-being and longevity. The demands of our work, the level of satisfaction and engagement we experience, and the lifestyle choices they engender collectively play a significant role in determining the quality and length of our lives. This comprehensive exploration will delve into the complex relationship between career choices and longevity, encompassing the impact of harmful career choices, the ways supportive choices can foster a long and healthy life, and strategies for making the most of your current career to optimize your well-being.

The trajectory of our careers is intricately woven into the fabric of our lives, influencing not only our financial well-being but also our mental, emotional, and physical health. While our work can provide purpose, a sense of accomplishment, and personal growth, it can also give rise to stress, burnout, and lifestyle choices that compromise our longevity. The choices we make regarding our careers hold the potential to shape the duration and quality of our lives. This comprehensive guide aims to explore the multifaceted relationship between career choices and longevity, offering insights into harmful choices, supportive strategies, and the art of harmonizing career pursuits with a healthy and fulfilling life.

THE DYNAMIC LINK BETWEEN CAREERS AND LONGEVITY

Our careers often form the cornerstone of our daily lives. The time, energy, and effort we invest in our work can have a significant impact on our well-being and longevity. The choices we make regarding our careers influence our stress levels, lifestyle habits, and overall life satisfaction.

HARMFUL CAREER CHOICES AND THEIR IMPACT ON LONGEVITY

Certain career choices can inadvertently contribute to stress, sedentary behavior, and detrimental habits that negatively impact longevity.

Chronic Stress and Burnout

High-stress jobs that demand long hours and constant availability can lead to chronic stress and burnout. The relentless pressure and lack of adequate time for relaxation and self-care can take a toll on physical and mental health. Chronic stress has been linked to increased risk of heart disease, immune suppression, and mental health disorders.

Sedentary Lifestyle and Physical Health

Sedentary jobs that involve prolonged periods of sitting can contribute to a sedentary lifestyle. The lack of movement and physical activity is associated with obesity, cardiovascular diseases, and musculoskeletal issues. Sitting for extended periods also negatively affects metabolism and blood circulation.

Unhealthy Habits and Work-Life Imbalance

Hectic work schedules and long hours can lead to poor lifestyle choices, including unhealthy eating habits, lack of exercise, and inadequate sleep. Balancing work and personal life becomes challenging, resulting in work-life imbalance that impacts overall well-being.

SUPPORTIVE CAREER CHOICES FOR A LONG AND HEALTHY LIFE

While certain career choices can be detrimental, others offer opportunities to promote well-being, personal growth, and a long and healthy life.

FULFILLING AND MEANINGFUL WORK

Engaging in work that aligns with your passions, values, and strengths can contribute to a sense of purpose and fulfillment. When your career is a source of joy and satisfaction, it positively impacts your mental and emotional well-being, reducing stress and promoting longevity.

Work-Life Integration and Balance

Choosing a career that values work-life integration and supports a balanced lifestyle is essential for long-term well-being. Flexible work arrangements, such as remote work options or flexible hours, allow you to prioritize health, family, and personal pursuits.

Opportunities for Growth and Learning

Opting for a career that offers opportunities for continuous learning and growth can foster a sense of accomplishment and intellectual stimulation. Embracing challenges and expanding your skill set can enhance self-esteem and contribute to a fulfilling life.

Strategies for Making the Most of Your Current Career

Whether you're navigating a fulfilling career or facing challenges in your current job, there are strategies to optimize your well-being within the context of your career.

Prioritizing Self-Care

No matter your career, prioritizing self-care is essential. Regular exercise, nutritious eating, sufficient sleep, and stress-reduction practices can mitigate the negative effects of a demanding job.

Cultivating Positive Relationships at Work

Building positive relationships with colleagues and supervisors creates a supportive and enjoyable work environment. Positive social connections contribute to emotional well-being and job satisfaction.

Embracing Lifelong Learning

Continuously seek opportunities for learning and skill development, even within your current role. Engaging in training programs, workshops, and online courses can boost your confidence and enhance your career prospects.

Navigating Transitions with Resilience

If you're considering a career transition, approach it with resilience and adaptability. Embrace change as an opportunity for growth, and leverage your existing skills and experiences to navigate new challenges.

The Role of Mindset and Attitude

Mindset and attitude play a pivotal role in how you experience your career and its impact on your longevity.

Finding Purpose and Satisfaction

Cultivating a positive mindset involves finding purpose and satisfaction in your career. Viewing your work as meaningful and understanding its contribution to your personal and professional growth can enhance your overall well-being.

Embracing Change and Adaptation

Adapting to the evolving landscape of your career requires a growth mindset. Embrace change as a chance to develop new skills, gain new perspectives, and open doors to opportunities you may not have considered before.

Balancing Long-Term Goals and Immediate Demands

Balancing long-term career aspirations with immediate demands is a delicate art that impacts both your career trajectory and well-being.

Nurturing Well-Being Amidst Ambitions

While setting ambitious career goals is commendable, it's crucial to nurture your well-being along the way. Prioritize stress management, self-care, and healthy habits to sustain your energy and motivation.

Making Time for Health and Relationships

Integrating health-promoting activities and nurturing relationships into your busy schedule is vital. Block out time for exercise, relaxation, and quality time with loved ones to maintain a holistic approach to well-being.

THE IMPORTANCE OF FINANCIAL HEALTH AND PLANNING

Financial health and planning have a significant impact on your career choices and overall well-being.

SECURING YOUR FUTURE AND REDUCING STRESS

Safeguarding your financial well-being through savings, investments, and appropriate insurance can reduce stress and provide a sense of security, allowing you to focus on your career and life goals.

BUILDING A BRIDGE TO RETIREMENT

Consider how your career choices align with your long-term retirement goals. Planning for retirement and gradually transitioning to less demanding roles can ensure a smooth transition from full-time work to a more relaxed pace.

CREATING A HOLISTIC APPROACH TO CAREER AND LONGEVITY

Achieving a harmonious balance between career ambitions and well-being requires a holistic approach.

INTEGRATING CAREER AND LIFESTYLE GOALS

Align your career choices with your overall lifestyle goals. Consider how your work enhances your life and enables you to pursue your passions and interests outside of the workplace.

PRIORITIZING PERSONAL FULFILLMENT

Ultimately, the success of your career is intertwined with your personal fulfillment and well-being. Prioritize your happiness and overall quality of life, making choices that contribute positively to both.

CONCLUSION

The relationship between career choices and longevity is intricate and multifaceted, reflecting the interplay between professional pursuits and personal well-being. Recognizing the potential impact of your career on your health empowers you to make informed choices that align with your values, aspirations, and overall life satisfaction. By selecting a career that supports your well-being, managing stress, and fostering positive relationships, you pave the way for a long, fulfilling, and healthy life. With mindful consideration, resilience, and an integrative approach, you can navigate your career journey in a manner that enriches your existence and contributes to a legacy of well-lived years.

Chapter 6: Financial Planning for Longer Living

In an era where life expectancy is increasing, financial planning takes on an even greater significance. As we aspire to live longer, healthier lives, it becomes imperative to ensure that our financial resources align with these aspirations.

Financial planning goes beyond mere budgeting; it encompasses strategies that safeguard our economic well-being, support our lifestyle choices, and provide us with the means to thrive throughout our extended years. This comprehensive guide will delve into the intricate realm of financial planning for a longer life, covering essential aspects such as retirement savings, investments, healthcare costs, estate planning, and sustainable financial habits.

As our understanding of health, wellness, and longevity continues to evolve, it is vital that our financial planning evolves alongside it. Financial planning for a longer life encompasses a comprehensive strategy that considers both our short-term needs and our long-term aspirations. It empowers us to align our financial decisions with our life goals, ensuring that we can not only sustain our lifestyle but also thrive as we age.

Understanding the Longevity Challenge

The prospect of living longer presents both opportunities and challenges. While the gift of extended years allows for more time to pursue passions and dreams, it also requires careful consideration of financial resources. Longer life spans mean increased healthcare expenses, extended retirement periods, and the need to ensure that our financial nest egg can withstand the test of time.

RETIREMENT PLANNING: NAVIGATING THE PATH TO FINANCIAL FREEDOM

Retirement planning is at the core of financial preparation for a longer life. It involves mapping out your financial journey to ensure a comfortable and secure retirement.

ASSESSING RETIREMENT NEEDS

Calculating your retirement needs involves estimating the funds required to maintain your desired lifestyle throughout your retirement years. Consider factors such as housing costs, healthcare expenses, travel, and leisure activities. An accurate assessment forms the foundation of your retirement savings goals.

DIVERSIFYING RETIREMENT INCOME

Relying solely on traditional pension plans might not be sufficient in today's dynamic economic landscape. Diversifying your retirement income sources can provide stability and reduce risk. Social Security benefits, pension plans, personal savings, and other investments collectively contribute to your retirement income.

MAXIMIZING RETIREMENT ACCOUNTS

Contributing to retirement accounts, such as 401(k)s, IRAs, and Roth IRAs, offers tax advantages and compounds your savings over time. Take advantage of employer-sponsored plans and explore options that align with your financial goals.

INVESTMENT STRATEGIES FOR LONG-TERM FINANCIAL SECURITY

Investing wisely is crucial for preserving and growing your wealth over the years.

EMBRACING DIVERSIFICATION

Diversifying your investment portfolio across different asset classes—such as stocks, bonds, real estate, and alternative investments—reduces risk and enhances potential returns. A diversified portfolio is better positioned to weather market fluctuations.

BALANCING RISK AND RETURN

Balancing risk and return is a fundamental principle of investing. While seeking higher returns can be enticing, it's essential to assess your risk tolerance and invest in alignment with your comfort level. Conservative investments may provide stability, while riskier ventures could yield higher rewards.

INVESTING IN HEALTH AND WELLNESS

As you plan for a longer life, consider investments in health and wellness. Prioritize activities, products, and services that contribute to your well-being. This includes maintaining a healthy lifestyle, exploring preventive healthcare, and investing in technologies that support aging in place.

ADDRESSING HEALTHCARE COSTS AND LONG-TERM CARE

Healthcare expenses are a significant consideration in financial planning for longevity.

ESTIMATING HEALTHCARE EXPENSES

Estimate your healthcare costs based on current health status and potential medical needs in the future. Consider premiums, deductibles, copays, and out-of-pocket expenses for medical services and prescription medications.

LONG-TERM CARE OPTIONS

Long-term care refers to assistance with daily activities for individuals with chronic illnesses, disabilities, or cognitive impairments. Explore long-term care insurance and other options to protect yourself from the potentially substantial costs associated with assisted living, nursing homes, or home care.

HEALTH SAVINGS ACCOUNTS (HSAS)
HSAs offer a tax-advantaged way to save for medical expenses. Contributions are tax-deductible, earnings grow tax-free, and withdrawals for qualified medical expenses are tax-free. HSAs provide a powerful tool for managing healthcare costs in retirement.

ESTATE PLANNING: ENSURING A LASTING LEGACY

Estate planning ensures that your assets are distributed according to your wishes and minimizes potential conflicts among beneficiaries.

WILLS AND TRUSTS
Drafting a will is a fundamental step in estate planning. It outlines how your assets will be distributed upon your passing. Trusts offer additional flexibility and control over asset distribution, often providing tax advantages.

NAMING BENEFICIARIES
Ensuring that your beneficiary designations are up-to-date on retirement accounts, insurance policies, and other assets is essential. Beneficiary designations override instructions in a will, so it's crucial to review them periodically.

CHARITABLE GIVING
Incorporating charitable giving into your estate plan allows you to leave a legacy aligned with your values. Charitable contributions can also have tax benefits for your heirs.

BUDGETING AND SUSTAINABLE FINANCIAL HABITS FOR LONGEVITY

Creating a sustainable budget and practicing prudent financial habits lay the groundwork for financial security.

CREATING A LONGEVITY-FOCUSED BUDGET
Design a budget that considers potential longevity-related expenses. Allocate funds for healthcare, leisure activities, and

potential long-term care needs. Monitor and adjust your budget as circumstances evolve.

Managing Debt

Managing and reducing debt is crucial for financial stability in retirement. Prioritize paying off high-interest debt, and consider downsizing or refinancing if necessary.

Cultivating Financial Resilience

Financial resilience involves building an emergency fund to handle unexpected expenses. Having a safety net ensures that unforeseen financial setbacks do not jeopardize your long-term plans.

Adapting to Changing Circumstances

Flexibility is essential in financial planning for longevity.

Flexibility in Financial Planning

Recognize that life is dynamic, and circumstances may change. Regularly review your financial plan and make adjustments as needed to accommodate evolving goals, market conditions, and economic shifts.

Navigating Economic Shifts

Economic downturns and market fluctuations are inevitable. Ensure that your investment portfolio is diversified and positioned to weather these shifts. Avoid making impulsive decisions driven by short-term market volatility.

Collaborating with Financial Professionals

Financial planning for a longer life benefits from the guidance of experts.

Seeking Expert Guidance

Consulting with financial advisors, estate planners, and tax professionals can provide insights tailored to your specific circumstances. These experts can help you make informed decisions aligned with your long-term goals.

MONITORING AND ADJUSTING PLANS

Regularly review your financial plan with professionals and make necessary adjustments. Life events, changes in the economy, and shifts in personal goals may warrant modifications to your plan.

CONCLUSION

Financial planning for a longer life is a multifaceted journey that intertwines financial well-being with the pursuit of longevity. It requires thoughtful consideration of retirement goals, investment strategies, healthcare costs, estate planning, and sustainable financial habits. As we aspire to embrace the potential of a longer life, strategic financial planning empowers us to make choices that support our well-being, provide economic security, and ensure that we can thrive throughout our extended years. By navigating this journey with prudence, flexibility, and the guidance of experts, we can create a financial landscape that aligns with our aspirations and enables us to enjoy the full richness of our extended lives.

Chapter 7: Relationships and Longevity

In the tapestry of life, relationships are the threads that weave together our experiences, emotions, and well-being. As we embark on a journey toward a long and healthy life, the quality of our relationships plays a pivotal role. From intimate partnerships and family connections to friendships and social networks, relationships offer support, companionship, and a sense of belonging that deeply influence our physical, mental, and emotional health. This comprehensive exploration will delve into the profound impact of relationships on longevity, encompassing the science behind social connections, fostering healthy relationships, overcoming challenges, and cultivating a vibrant social support system for a fulfilling life.

The journey toward a long and healthy life is enriched when shared with others. Relationships, whether intimate or platonic, familial or friendly, are the threads that weave a vibrant tapestry of experiences. Human beings are inherently social creatures, and the connections we form play an integral role in our overall well-being. In an era marked by technological advancement and fast-paced living, understanding the profound impact of relationships on our longevity becomes even more crucial.

The Science of Social Connections and Longevity

Scientific research has illuminated the intricate relationship between social connections and longevity.

The Longevity Paradox

While individual lifestyle choices, such as diet and exercise, significantly influence health and longevity, research reveals that social connections play an equally crucial role. In fact, studies consistently demonstrate that strong social ties are associated with a reduced risk of mortality and better health outcomes.

THE LONELINESS EPIDEMIC

Conversely, loneliness and social isolation have been linked to adverse health effects. Loneliness can elevate stress hormones, increase inflammation, and weaken the immune system. As a result, individuals who lack meaningful connections are at a higher risk of developing chronic diseases and experiencing premature mortality.

HEALTHY RELATIONSHIPS: THE CORNERSTONE OF WELL-BEING

Healthy relationships contribute to emotional resilience, stress reduction, and overall well-being.

INTIMATE PARTNERSHIPS AND THEIR IMPACT

Intimate partnerships provide emotional support, companionship, and a safe space for vulnerability. A nurturing partnership can reduce stress, boost happiness, and provide a sense of purpose and fulfillment.

FAMILY CONNECTIONS AND THEIR INFLUENCE

Family relationships offer a unique blend of support, history, and shared experiences. Positive family dynamics can provide a sense of belonging and a safety net in times of need.

THE POWER OF FRIENDSHIPS

Friendships provide a valuable avenue for companionship, shared interests, and emotional connection. Strong friendships enhance mental well-being, lower stress levels, and even encourage healthier lifestyle habits.

BUILDING AND SUSTAINING SOCIAL NETWORKS

Cultivating a diverse social network allows for a rich tapestry of interactions. Engaging with various circles, from work colleagues to community groups, provides opportunities for learning, growth, and the exchange of ideas.

NAVIGATING RELATIONSHIP CHALLENGES FOR LONGEVITY

Healthy relationships require effort, communication, and a commitment to growth.

Communication and Conflict Resolution

Effective communication is the cornerstone of healthy relationships. Open dialogues, active listening, and the ability to resolve conflicts constructively strengthen connections and minimize misunderstandings.

Embracing Change and Growth

Relationships evolve over time, and embracing growth is essential. Supporting each other's personal development and adapting to changing circumstances contribute to the longevity of relationships.

Addressing Isolation and Loneliness

In a hyperconnected world, feelings of isolation can still persist. Combat loneliness by proactively seeking out social interactions, participating in group activities, and fostering connections online and offline.

Cultivating a Vibrant Social Support System

Cultivating a robust social support system involves intentional efforts.

Prioritizing Meaningful Interactions

Quality trumps quantity when it comes to social connections. Prioritize meaningful interactions that provide emotional resonance, understanding, and a sense of belonging.

Quality vs. Quantity in Relationships

Having a few close, trusted relationships can be more impactful than a large network of superficial connections. Quality relationships offer deeper emotional support and companionship.

Embracing Diversity in Relationships

Diversity in relationships fosters personal growth and expands perspectives. Engage with people of different ages, backgrounds, and interests to enrich your social tapestry.

THE CONNECTION BETWEEN RELATIONSHIPS AND MENTAL HEALTH

Relationships significantly influence mental health and resilience.

MITIGATING STRESS AND ANXIETY

Strong social ties serve as buffers against stress and anxiety. Social support systems provide outlets for sharing concerns and receiving empathy, alleviating emotional burdens.

FOSTERING RESILIENCE THROUGH CONNECTIONS

Navigating life's challenges is made easier with a strong support system. Relationships offer encouragement, advice, and a source of strength during difficult times.

THE ROLE OF RELATIONSHIPS IN PHYSICAL HEALTH AND LONGEVITY

The impact of relationships extends beyond mental well-being to physical health.

HEART HEALTH AND SOCIAL BONDS

Positive relationships are associated with improved heart health. The emotional support provided by loved ones helps manage stress and contributes to cardiovascular well-being.

IMMUNE SYSTEM BOOST FROM SOCIAL CONNECTIONS

A robust social support system enhances immune system function. Meaningful connections trigger the release of positive hormones that contribute to overall health.

AGING TOGETHER: RELATIONSHIPS IN LATER LIFE

The dynamics of relationships shift as we age, and nurturing connections becomes even more vital.

Redefining Roles and Dynamics

As children grow and leave the nest, couples must redefine their roles and find new ways to connect. This phase of life offers an opportunity to rediscover each other and embrace shared interests.

Supporting One Another Through Aging

As we age, the importance of relationships grows. Friends and family provide companionship, assistance, and emotional support during the challenges of aging.

The Impact of Digital Relationships

Digital connections have reshaped the landscape of relationships.

Navigating Virtual Connections

Online interactions can provide companionship and connection, especially for individuals with limited mobility. Virtual friendships can be meaningful, but striking a balance between virtual and in-person connections is essential.

Balancing Virtual and In-Person Interactions

While digital connections have their benefits, the richness of in-person interactions remains unparalleled. Prioritize face-to-face connections to fully experience the emotional depth of relationships.

Conclusion

In the journey toward a long and healthy life, relationships stand as the foundation upon which we build our experiences, emotions, and well-being. The depth of our connections profoundly influences our mental, emotional, and physical health. As we navigate the complexities of life, nurturing relationships, cultivating meaningful interactions, and fostering a vibrant social support system become essential elements in our pursuit of longevity. By recognizing the power of relationships, embracing growth, and valuing both in-person and digital connections, we weave a tapestry of companionship, understanding, and joy that enriches every facet of our journey toward a fulfilling and extended life.

Chapter 8: Partners in Longevity

In the pursuit of a long and healthy life, our professional allies play a crucial role in guiding us toward well-being, offering expert advice, and providing the tools needed to make informed decisions. From healthcare professionals and nutritionists to fitness trainers and therapists, enlisting the expertise of professionals can significantly impact our physical, mental, and emotional health. This chapter explores the array of professionals who contribute to our well-being, detailing their roles, the benefits they offer, and how their guidance can be seamlessly integrated into our pursuit of longevity.

The journey toward a long and healthy life is a multidimensional endeavor, requiring a holistic approach that addresses physical, mental, emotional, and even financial well-being. Professionals in various fields possess specialized knowledge that can significantly contribute to our pursuit of longevity. By enlisting their guidance, we can tap into a wealth of expertise that supports our well-being and empowers us to make informed decisions aligned with our aspirations for a fulfilling and extended life.

Healthcare Professionals: Navigating Physical Well-Being

Healthcare professionals serve as the frontline defenders of our physical health.

Physicians and Primary Care Providers

Primary care physicians play a pivotal role in preventive care and early detection of health issues. Regular check-ups, screenings, and immunizations are essential components of their guidance.

Specialists and Subspecialists

Specialists provide expert insights into specific health conditions. Subspecialists offer specialized care within these fields. Whether it's cardiology, dermatology, or orthopedics, their expertise helps manage complex health concerns.

NURSES AND NURSE PRACTITIONERS

Nurses are instrumental in patient care, providing support, administering treatments, and offering education. Nurse practitioners often have advanced training, enabling them to diagnose and treat certain conditions.

PHARMACISTS

Pharmacists offer medication expertise, ensuring proper dosages, interactions, and potential side effects. They play a critical role in medication management, particularly for those with chronic conditions.

NUTRITIONISTS AND DIETITIANS: FUELING LONGEVITY THROUGH NUTRITION

Nutritionists and dietitians guide us toward optimal eating habits.

ASSESSING NUTRITIONAL NEEDS

These professionals assess individual nutritional needs based on factors such as age, activity level, and health status. They tailor dietary recommendations to support overall health and specific goals.

TAILORING DIETARY PLANS

Nutritionists create customized meal plans that address dietary restrictions, weight management, and health objectives. They help individuals make healthier food choices that align with their well-being goals.

SUPPORTING LIFESTYLE CHANGES

By offering practical strategies, education, and ongoing support, nutritionists empower individuals to adopt sustainable eating habits that contribute to longevity and well-being.

FITNESS TRAINERS: BUILDING PHYSICAL RESILIENCE

Fitness trainers guide us on the path to physical vitality.

CUSTOMIZED EXERCISE PROGRAMS

Fitness trainers design exercise routines tailored to individual goals, abilities, and preferences. These programs encompass cardiovascular, strength training, flexibility, and balance exercises.

MOTIVATION AND ACCOUNTABILITY

Trainers provide motivation and accountability, which are crucial for maintaining an active lifestyle. They offer guidance, track progress, and adjust routines to prevent plateaus and boredom.

PREVENTING INJURIES AND OVERTRAINING

Trainers ensure proper form and technique, reducing the risk of injuries. They also help individuals strike a balance between challenging workouts and avoiding overtraining.

MENTAL HEALTH PROFESSIONALS: CULTIVATING EMOTIONAL RESILIENCE

Mental health professionals nurture emotional well-being and resilience.

PSYCHOLOGISTS AND THERAPISTS

Psychologists and therapists offer talk therapy and counseling, addressing a range of emotional and mental health concerns. They provide coping strategies, stress management techniques, and tools for personal growth.

PSYCHIATRISTS

Psychiatrists are medical doctors specializing in mental health. They can diagnose and treat mental illnesses, often prescribing medication to support emotional well-being.

COUNSELORS AND SOCIAL WORKERS

Counselors and social workers provide counseling and support for individuals and families facing challenges such as relationship issues, grief, or major life transitions.

FINANCIAL ADVISORS: SECURING ECONOMIC WELL-BEING

Financial advisors guide us in creating a secure financial foundation for longevity.

RETIREMENT AND FINANCIAL PLANNING

Financial advisors help develop retirement savings plans that align with long-term goals. They consider factors such as retirement age, lifestyle preferences, and healthcare costs.

LONG-TERM CARE PLANNING

Advisors offer insights into funding options for potential long-term care needs. They help individuals prepare for potential expenses associated with aging and healthcare.

ESTATE PLANNING

Estate planning ensures that assets are distributed according to individual wishes. Advisors assist in creating wills, trusts, and designating beneficiaries to secure a lasting legacy.

CAREER COACHES: BALANCING PROFESSIONAL ASPIRATIONS AND WELL-BEING

Career coaches assist in aligning professional pursuits with overall well-being.

ALIGNING CAREER CHOICES WITH LIFESTYLE GOALS

Career coaches help individuals identify opportunities that align with their values, skills, and long-term aspirations. They provide guidance on making career choices that promote work-life balance.

NAVIGATING TRANSITIONS AND BURNOUT

Coaches offer support during career transitions, whether it's changing fields, seeking promotions, or reentering the workforce after a hiatus. They help prevent burnout by teaching stress management techniques.

PRIORITIZING WORK-LIFE BALANCE

Work-life balance is essential for longevity. Career coaches guide individuals in negotiating flexible arrangements, setting boundaries, and integrating self-care into their routines.

HOLISTIC HEALTH PRACTITIONERS: INTEGRATING MIND, BODY, AND SPIRIT

Holistic health practitioners approach well-being from a comprehensive perspective.

INTEGRATIVE MEDICINE PHYSICIANS

Integrative medicine practitioners combine conventional medical approaches with complementary therapies. They consider physical, emotional, and spiritual aspects of health when creating treatment plans.

ACUPUNCTURISTS AND TRADITIONAL HEALERS

These practitioners offer alternative therapies that promote balance and well-being. Acupuncture, herbal medicine, and other modalities can contribute to overall vitality.

MINDFULNESS COACHES

Mindfulness coaches teach techniques for cultivating present-moment awareness and reducing stress. Mindfulness practices enhance mental clarity, emotional regulation, and overall well-being.

TECHNOLOGY EXPERTS: LEVERAGING INNOVATION FOR HEALTH

Technology experts harness digital tools for health and well-being.

TELEHEALTH PROFESSIONALS

Telehealth professionals provide medical consultations and mental health support through virtual platforms. This accessibility enhances healthcare access, particularly for those with mobility constraints.

HEALTH AND WELLNESS APPS

Wellness apps offer tools for tracking nutrition, exercise, sleep, and stress levels. These apps facilitate self-care, goal-setting, and staying accountable to health objectives.

WEARABLE TECHNOLOGY AND HEALTH TRACKING

Wearable devices monitor physical activity, heart rate, sleep patterns, and more. They provide real-time data that informs lifestyle choices and empowers individuals to make healthier decisions.

COLLABORATIVE APPROACH: INTEGRATING PROFESSIONAL GUIDANCE FOR LONGEVITY

The synergy of various professionals fosters comprehensive well-being.

COORDINATING CARE ACROSS PROFESSIONALS

When facing complex health concerns, coordinating care among different professionals ensures a holistic approach. This collaboration results in integrated treatment plans.

CREATING A PERSONALIZED WELL-BEING TEAM

Building a team of professionals that aligns with individual goals maximizes well-being efforts. Each professional contributes unique insights to support overall health.

CONCLUSION

The journey toward a long and healthy life is an intricate tapestry woven together by the expertise of professionals who contribute to our well-being. From healthcare and nutrition to fitness, mental health, finances, and career choices, these professionals serve as valuable allies on our path to longevity. By harnessing their guidance, integrating their recommendations, and adopting a collaborative approach to well-being, we empower ourselves to make informed choices that enhance our quality of life, resilience, and overall vitality.

Chapter 9: Goal Setting

In the pursuit of a long and healthy life, setting meaningful goals becomes a cornerstone of success. Goals provide direction, purpose, and a roadmap for the choices we make each day. As we navigate the complexities of modern living, intentional goal setting empowers us to align our actions with our aspirations for longevity. This comprehensive exploration will delve into the art and science of goal setting for a long and healthy life, encompassing the psychology of goals, creating a holistic goal framework, overcoming obstacles, and the transformative impact of goal achievement on our well-being.

Goal setting serves as a compass, guiding us toward a long and healthy life filled with purpose and well-being. In a world replete with distractions and demands, deliberate goal setting empowers us to take charge of our destiny and make choices that align with our aspirations for a fulfilling and extended life. By understanding the psychology of goals, crafting a holistic goal framework, overcoming challenges, and experiencing the transformative impact of achievement, we unlock the potential to live a life that thrives on intentionality and purpose.

Understanding the Psychology of Goal Setting

The psychology of goal setting reveals the intricate relationship between our aspirations, actions, and well-being.

The Power of Purpose

Setting goals provides a sense of purpose that propels us forward. Purpose-driven individuals tend to exhibit greater resilience, happiness, and overall well-being.

SMART Goals: Specific, Measurable, Achievable, Relevant, Time-Bound

The SMART framework guides effective goal setting. Goals should be Specific (clear and well-defined), Measurable (quantifiable), Achievable (realistic), Relevant (aligned with values), and Time-Bound (with a clear timeframe).

Intrinsic vs. Extrinsic Motivation

Goals are fueled by either intrinsic (internal) or extrinsic (external) motivation. Intrinsic motivation, driven by personal enjoyment and satisfaction, often leads to more sustainable goal pursuit and greater well-being outcomes.

Crafting Holistic Goals for Longevity

Holistic goals encompass various dimensions of well-being, creating a balanced approach to a long and healthy life.

Physical Well-Being Goals

Physical goals focus on aspects such as fitness, nutrition, sleep, and preventive healthcare. Examples include achieving a certain level of physical activity, maintaining a balanced diet, and getting adequate sleep.

Mental and Emotional Well-Being Goals

Mental and emotional goals prioritize psychological health. Examples include practicing mindfulness, managing stress effectively, cultivating positive self-talk, and seeking therapy when needed.

Social and Relationship Goals

Social goals revolve around building and nurturing meaningful connections. Examples include strengthening relationships, expanding social networks, and contributing positively to the community.

Financial and Career Goals

Financial and career goals ensure economic stability and fulfillment. Examples include saving for retirement, pursuing a meaningful career, and aligning professional choices with personal values.

Personal Growth and Lifelong Learning Goals

Personal growth goals encompass continuous learning and self-improvement. Examples include acquiring new skills, pursuing hobbies, and exploring personal passions.

OVERCOMING CHALLENGES AND OBSTACLES

While goal pursuit is rewarding, challenges and obstacles are inevitable.

OVERCOMING PROCRASTINATION

Procrastination hinders goal achievement. Strategies such as breaking goals into smaller tasks, setting deadlines, and using accountability mechanisms help overcome this hurdle.

NAVIGATING SETBACKS AND FAILURES

Setbacks and failures are part of any journey. Resilience is key to bouncing back from challenges. Viewing setbacks as learning opportunities and adjusting goals as needed supports continued progress.

SUSTAINING MOTIVATION AND MOMENTUM

Maintaining motivation over the long haul requires strategies such as visualization, positive self-affirmations, and regularly revisiting the reasons behind your goals.

THE TRANSFORMATIVE IMPACT OF GOAL ACHIEVEMENT

Achieving goals goes beyond the tangible outcomes; it profoundly affects our well-being.

BOOSTING SELF-ESTEEM AND CONFIDENCE

Goal achievement enhances self-esteem and confidence. Accomplishing what we set out to do validates our abilities and reinforces our sense of self-worth.

ENHANCING MENTAL AND EMOTIONAL RESILIENCE

Navigating challenges during goal pursuit fosters emotional resilience. The process of overcoming obstacles builds coping skills and emotional strength.

FOSTERING A SENSE OF PURPOSE AND FULFILLMENT

Attaining goals contributes to a sense of purpose and fulfillment. Accomplishments align with our values, creating a meaningful narrative for our lives.

Integrating Goal Setting into Daily Life

Incorporating goal setting into our daily routines ensures consistent progress.

Setting Short-Term and Long-Term Goals

Balancing short-term and long-term goals allows for steady progress while maintaining a sense of urgency and accomplishment.

Prioritizing and Time Management

Effective time management is essential for goal attainment. Prioritize tasks, allocate time wisely, and minimize distractions to stay on track.

Celebrating Milestones and Progress

Celebrate milestones and progress to stay motivated. Acknowledging even small achievements provides positive reinforcement and sustains momentum.

Goal Setting as a Lifelong Journey

Goal setting is not a one-time event but a dynamic and ongoing process.

Evolving Goals as Priorities Shift

As life evolves, our priorities change. Regularly reassess goals and adjust them to align with changing circumstances and aspirations.

Embracing Adaptability and Flexibility

Flexibility is essential in goal pursuit. Unexpected challenges and opportunities arise, and adapting our goals allows us to seize these moments.

Conclusion

Goal setting is the thread that weaves intentionality into the fabric of our lives. In the pursuit of a long and healthy life, deliberate goal setting empowers us to navigate challenges, embrace opportunities, and align our actions with our aspirations. By understanding the psychology of goals, crafting a holistic framework, overcoming obstacles, and reaping the transformative rewards of achievement, we embark on a journey enriched with purpose, well-being, and the fulfillment that arises from living a life driven by intention and guided by goals.

Chapter 10: Making Your Plan for Longevity

In the pursuit of a long and healthy life, a personalized plan serves as a guiding light, illuminating the steps, choices, and strategies that align with your unique aspirations. Each individual's journey is a mosaic of physical, mental, emotional, and social dimensions, interwoven with diverse goals and priorities. This comprehensive guide will navigate the intricate process of developing a tailored plan for longevity, encompassing self-assessment, goal identification, lifestyle adjustments, habit formation, and the power of ongoing self-care.

Crafting an individualized plan for a long and healthy life is an empowering journey that honors your unique attributes, values, and goals. In a world of myriad influences and demands, developing a personalized roadmap ensures that your choices and actions harmonize with your aspirations for a vibrant and extended life. By embarking on this journey of self-discovery, setting meaningful goals, making sustainable lifestyle adjustments, nurturing habits, and prioritizing ongoing self-care, you create a profound framework that enriches your journey toward longevity.

The Art of Self-Assessment

Self-assessment is the cornerstone of a personalized longevity plan.

Reflecting on Current Lifestyle

Honest self-reflection allows you to evaluate your current habits, routines, and choices. Identifying patterns that either support or hinder your well-being forms the basis for meaningful change.

Identifying Strengths and Areas for Improvement

Celebrate your strengths while acknowledging areas that need improvement. This holistic view provides a balanced perspective for crafting your plan.

SETTING CLEAR INTENTIONS
Establish a clear intention for your longevity journey. This intention will serve as a guiding principle that informs every decision you make moving forward.

SETTING HOLISTIC LONGEVITY GOALS

Holistic goals address all dimensions of well-being.

DEFINING PHYSICAL WELL-BEING GOALS
Physical goals encompass aspects such as fitness, nutrition, sleep, and preventive healthcare. These goals ensure that your body is equipped for vitality and resilience.

CULTIVATING MENTAL AND EMOTIONAL RESILIENCE GOALS
Mental and emotional goals focus on psychological well-being. Strategies for managing stress, fostering positivity, and nurturing emotional intelligence contribute to mental resilience.

FOSTERING SOCIAL CONNECTION AND RELATIONSHIP GOALS
Social and relationship goals emphasize the importance of nurturing connections with loved ones and expanding your social network. These connections are vital for emotional support and a sense of belonging.

NURTURING FINANCIAL, CAREER, AND PERSONAL GROWTH GOALS
Financial and career goals provide economic stability and fulfillment. Personal growth goals encourage continuous learning, skill development, and pursuing passions.

CREATING LIFESTYLE ADJUSTMENTS

Lifestyle adjustments lay the foundation for longevity.

BALANCING NUTRITION AND HYDRATION

Evaluate your dietary choices and make adjustments that align with your well-being goals. Prioritize whole foods, hydration, and mindful eating.

INCORPORATING PHYSICAL ACTIVITY
Regular physical activity supports cardiovascular health, strength, and flexibility. Choose activities you enjoy to ensure consistency and longevity.

PRIORITIZING SLEEP AND REST
Prioritize quality sleep for physical and mental rejuvenation. Develop a bedtime routine and create a sleep-conducive environment.

EMBRACING STRESS MANAGEMENT TECHNIQUES
Stress management is crucial for overall well-being. Incorporate relaxation techniques, mindfulness, and hobbies that bring joy and reduce stress.

THE SCIENCE OF HABIT FORMATION
Habit formation transforms intentions into actions.

UNDERSTANDING HABIT LOOPS AND TRIGGERS
Habits follow a loop of cue, routine, and reward. Identifying triggers and replacing negative routines with positive ones is key to habit change.

SETTING SMART GOALS FOR HABIT CHANGE
SMART goals (Specific, Measurable, Achievable, Relevant, Time-Bound) facilitate habit formation. Break down larger goals into smaller, manageable steps.

CONSISTENCY AND ACCOUNTABILITY IN HABIT FORMATION
Consistency is paramount for habit formation. Establish accountability mechanisms, such as tracking progress or partnering with a friend, to maintain momentum.

NURTURING ONGOING SELF-CARE

Ongoing self-care sustains your well-being journey.

THE ROLE OF MINDFULNESS AND MIND-BODY PRACTICES
Mindfulness practices enhance self-awareness, reduce stress, and foster emotional regulation. Incorporate meditation, deep breathing, and yoga into your routine.

PRACTICING GRATITUDE AND POSITIVE AFFIRMATIONS
Cultivate a positive mindset by practicing gratitude and using positive affirmations. These practices shift your focus toward the positive aspects of life.

SEEKING PROFESSIONAL SUPPORT AS NEEDED
Don't hesitate to seek professional support when necessary. Mental health professionals, nutritionists, and fitness trainers offer expert guidance on specific aspects of your plan.

ADAPTING TO LIFE'S CHANGES

Flexibility and adaptability ensure the longevity of your plan.

FLEXIBILITY AND RESILIENCE IN YOUR PLAN
Life is full of surprises and changes. Embrace adaptability as you navigate unexpected shifts, and adjust your plan accordingly.

EMBRACING AGING WITH GRACE AND ADAPTABILITY
As you age, your needs and priorities may change. Embrace the aging process with grace, adjusting your plan to align with your evolving aspirations.

CONCLUSION

Designing an individualized plan for a long and healthy life is a transformative journey that empowers you to take control of your well-being. By conducting a comprehensive self-assessment, setting holistic goals, making lifestyle adjustments, nurturing habits, and prioritizing ongoing self-care, you cultivate a foundation that supports longevity and fulfillment. This plan serves as a compass, guiding you through the complexities of modern life with intentionality, resilience, and the knowledge

that you are crafting a future that reflects your deepest
aspirations for a vibrant and extended journey.